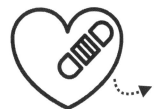  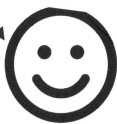

MW00413672

EMOTIONAL
WHOLENESS
CHECKLIST

ANDREW EDWIN JENKINS

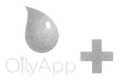
OllyApp +

A BOOK YOU'LL
ACTUALLY READ ABOUT
THE "FEELINGS KIT"

ISBN number = 9781793007698

Connect online!

Podcast-
OilyApp.com

Social-
www.Facebook.com/OilyApp
www.Facebook.com/OilyApp
www.Instagram.com/OilyApp

YouTube-
www.YouTube.com/Overflow

Website-
OilyApp.com
Jenkins.tv

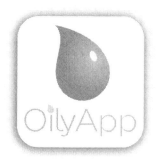

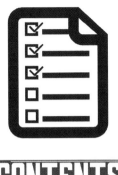

CONTENTS

AN OVERVIEW OF WHERE WE'RE HEADED!

INTRODUCTION

ABOUT THIS BOOK + ABOUT THIS SERIES

We created OilyApp (go to OilyApp.com to learn more) with the goal of educating you about Young Living's vast array of incredible products. The app is uniquely the *only* third party app that's an approved partner of Young Living Essential Oils, passing a strict compliance review each time we update.

OilyApp works well with Young Living's stated mission of taking oils into every home in the world. Once the oils get there, people need to know... *how do we use them?!*

Whereas shipping a desk reference to everyone is cumbersome and difficult (besides, who wants to always lug it around!?), most people have a smart phone. An app is the perfect solution.

Furthermore, the app was created by actual members (Ernie Yarbrough, one of the founders, and his wife are Royal Crown Diamonds). In other words, it was built in the field for use in the field.

THE NEXT THING

After a few years of providing users with OilyApp, it became apparent than another addition was needed for product users and business builders who wanted to go to the "next level." Enter OilyApp+, a web-based experience designed to provide users with more relevant information- things like scripts they could use to learn and/or educate their teams, graphics that were relevant and educational, and access to Diamond+ leaders.

We created OilyApp+ in less than two weeks from its conception.

From the beginning, we knew we wanted the OA+ to include video courses and online scripts- tools you could use to review and then teach your "people" what you were learning.

After a few weeks, the thought hit us: *What if we made the scripts into small books, too- small pocket-sized books people could easily review and use to study, to lead others, and even to teach classes?*

Hence the title you have in your hand.

The script and the videos where we teach the material are available in OA+ (access it all at OilyApp.com).

ABOUT THE EMOTIONAL CHECKLIST

Emotions are a big deal. Really big.

The problem is that we talk very little about them.

We've been told not to trust them, we've been accused of being "too emotional," and we've over-reacted just enough to prove the theory that we need to be less emotional correct.

We've also been told that some emotions are "good" and others are "bad." And we've been shunned for feeling those "taboo" ones too often while not feeling the good ones enough.

It all gets to be rather sticky and infinitely tricky, doesn't it?

In this short book, we'll talk about the"messy" world of feelings. You'll learn that...

- We're all emotional. Our emotions are a vital part of who we are (chapter 1).

- We can only be as healthy as the weakest part of us- be it our bodies, our minds, our spirits, or (yes!) our emotions. A more emotionally whole you is a healthier you (chapter 2).

- There are two things that help us transform into who we're designed to be spiritually and emotionally. You'll be surprised at what they are, and how accessible they are (chapter 3).

- Fear isn't a liar. Nor are any of your emotions. They're given to you as gifts to help you interpret what's happening around you and in you (chapter 4).

- Once we recognize our emotions, we can realize what they're communicating to us. Then, rather than being controlled by them, we can respond in a healthy way. We'll discuss this when we work through the Emotional Wholeness Checklist (chapter 5).

- Yes, we want to live in the present- and in the future- in an emotionally whole way. Sometimes, though, we need to go back in order to move ahead (chapter 6).

- Finally, we'll briefly talk through the Feelings Kit from Young Living Essential Oils. We'll learn how to use its six oils in conjunction with our Checklist (chapter 7).

LEAN IN + DIG DEEP

That said, don't be afraid of the "tough" or "bad" emotions. You'll learn there aren't good emotions and bad emotions- just "good" expressions and "bad" expressions of them.

My advice… is to lean in…

In *Emotionally Healthy Spirituality*, Peter Scazzero quotes Gerald Sitter's book *A Grace Disguised*:

> *The quickest way to reach the sun and the light of day is not to run west chasing after it, but to head east into the darkness until you finally reach the sunrise.*

We're often afraid of the dark. Not the physical dark, but the emotional dark. The silence. The quiet spaces.

Perhaps that's why we spend so much time on social media, mindlessly flipping and scrolling through our social feeds. In some sense, we're avoiding the dark. We're avoiding the hard spaces. We're chasing light and hope and anything to numb us.

The problem is, well, like the quote above suggests, if you move *towards* the sun, *towards* the warmth, you'll find yourself forever chasing the very thing that's moving away from you. The sun will remain just out of reach. It's only when we turn and move straight into the darkness, that cold bleakness that can seem so scary, that we find ourselves-

- No longer chasing the sun, *nor*

- No longer trying to outrun the hurts + pains of the past, *but also*

- Moving into the precise direction that will take us into the light most quickly and assuredly.

Let's flip the page and get to work!

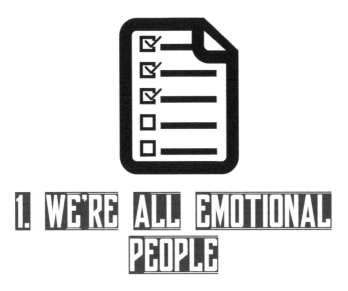

1. WE'RE ALL EMOTIONAL PEOPLE

MAIN IDEA= EMOTIONS ARE PART OF WHO WE ARE. IF WE DON'T FIND A HEALTHY WAY TO EXPRESS THEM, OUR FEELINGS "COME OUT" IN UNHEALTHY WAYS.

A few years ago I began meeting with a counselor. He tells me that his first impression of me was, "Wow. He's an expressive and emotional guy."

A few years before that a federal judge helped a nonprofit where I worked, helping people who were coming off the streets, leaving addictions, and transitioning from prison or jail. After sitting through a few meetings, her assessment was similar: "He communicates with heart and passion."

If you would have asked me if I was emotional, though, I would have responded with an emphatic, "No, I'm not!"

I've noticed a few things about myself, though, things that are likely true of most people:

- Passion and pain come from the same space inside of us. If you turn off "hurt" you automatically turn off joy. The two flow from the same facet, so to stop the flow of one is to prohibit the flow of the other.

- Both must be expressed- or the pressure "builds up inside the pipes."

In other words, we're all emotional. We can express it in a healthy way or- eventually- it builds up and spews out in some other manner.

I never had a filter to see pain as masculine. Or even Biblical. I remember being told not to cry multiple times throughout my childhood.

I didn't have a filter to see passion in that way, either. I remember being taunted for expressing myself passionately in worship, and I rarely saw strong men who also lived from an emotionally healthy center.

Since I closed off pain, I simultaneously shuddered joy and bliss. Yes, sometimes pieces of those emotions leaked. People like the counselor and the judge saw glimpses of the goldmine that was there. But, as you'll learn later in the book (chapter 6), it's easy to bury that stuff under a tough outer shell.

Nonetheless, these emotions *do* find a way to "leak out." They do so in moments when we're unguarded. Or, they do the only other thing they *can* do when you restrain them- *the emotional pipes burst!*

Let me explain…

EXPLODING EMOTIONS

One day a child-therapist with whom our family worked with described stress in a revealing way. Kristen, the counselor, likened our souls to balloons…

"You can blow a balloon up," she said, moving her hands larger and farther part as if an expanding party-type of balloon rested between them. "At first the balloon *is fine* with the air you blow in…"

She emphasized the word *fine*, highlighting that things were about to *not* be *fine*. Her hands continued moving further apart, demonstrating to us that the balloon between them was enlarging.

"At some point, the balloons reaches max capacity,' the continued. "Then we have four options."

She described the first three scenarios, explaining that-

- **First, you can continue adding air to the balloon, thereby causing it to pop.** This happens to some people. They- *seemingly overnight-* explode.[1] They "flip their lid." They lose it.

- **Second, you can squeak and squeal the balloon**, shrilling a sound that lets you know something is not right. I'm sure you've met people like this- people who seek to dominate tough situations by complaining, acting caustic, or exerting control over others.

---

1 It's never "overnight," though. Remember the straw that broke the camel's back is never the only straw.

- **Third, you can "let go" and watch the problem fly away**
  (read: hide).[2] People like this are the proverbial "take my toys and go home" pouters.

When my kids do *any of the three* with an actual balloon, I get equally anxious. The anticipation of the pop, the shrill, or the flying object is enough to drive me to the edge of the cliff alone.

Kristen didn't pop the balloon. She shrieked it. Yeah, she created that high-pitched fingers-on-chalkboard sound for a few moments. Then she let it go.

"That's how most people generally deal with stress," she said. "Rarely do people have the self-awareness to just step back and a do a **fourth option- that is, remove some of the air, and then let the balloon subsist at a comfortable level that maintains margin**."

"Seems like that would be the healthiest option," I said. "I've learned by now that there's always something going on, something which requires that margin."

FOUR WAYS TO COPE!

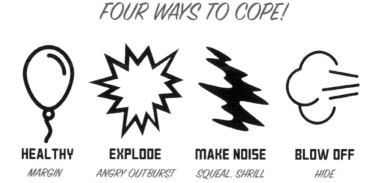

HEALTHY	EXPLODE	MAKE NOISE	BLOW OFF
MARGIN	*ANGRY OUTBURST*	*SQUEAL. SHRILL*	*HIDE*

2

I thought back through the past few years. Seems like we moved from one crisis to the next. I always thought something like, *when we get through this one, it will get better.*

Crisis seemed to be constant, though. We would get through one, have a week of ease, and then something else *always* came up. I thought it was just me. Turns out, it's like that for most people. A lot of people are struggling.

The irony is that, at the time I learned this from Kristen, I worked 60-80 hours a week. I tag-teamed carpooling to multiple therapies each week with Cristy, and we had the kids involved in sports. Oh, and she had just launched our essential oil business (which, in all honesty, became our financial life raft).

"You're living at your stress ceiling, your wife is operating at hers, and your son is clearly above his…"

I locked-on to something she said: "That balloon explodes and is done, it blows off and retreats to some random place, or it shrills and gets everyone's attention for the long haul…."

THE THREE UNHEALTHY OPTIONS LOOK LIKE...

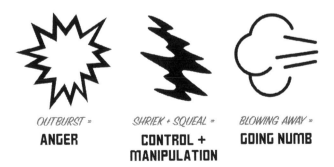

OUTBURST =	*SHRIEK + SQUEAL =*	*BLOWING AWAY =*
ANGER	**CONTROL + MANIPULATION**	**GOING NUMB**

The relational trends I've mentioned were already obvious-

Now, we were there to talk about some of our kids, but I received a lot of info about how adults operate. You see, a lot of us tend to exert control by shrilling (option 2).

MAKE CONSISTENT NOISE

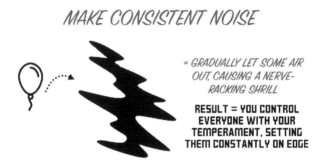

= GRADUALLY LET SOME AIR OUT, CAUSING A NERVE-RACKING SHRILL

RESULT = YOU CONTROL EVERYONE WITH YOUR TEMPERAMENT, SETTING THEM CONSTANTLY ON EDGE

This seems to be the *modus operandi* on social media. Face it: people say things on their social feeds about other people that they would never say in person.

I tend to do what most guys do- the other two options.

Let me be blunt. Guys generally do two things when it comes to emotionally responding (apart from doing it in a healthy way)-

- We get angry and explode (then expect normalcy the next day or sooner- after all, we got things off our chest and are OK now) (option 1).

- We go numb, generally making a bit of noise as we scurry off the scene. (we hide) (option 3).

Just like the balloon.

EXPLODING!

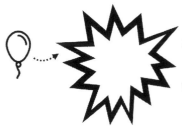

TOO MUCH PRESSURE =
THE BALLOON OVER-FILLS
& EXPLODES

RESULT = YOU FEEL LIKE
YOU DEALT WITH THE REAL
ISSUE, BUT YOU DIDN'T.
IT'S A TEMPORARY FIX.

BLOW OFF

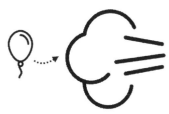

= LET GO OF THE BALLOON
IMMEDIATELY- THE AIR LEAVES,
THE BALLOON FLIES OFF

RESULT = KINDER THAN AN
ANGRY OUTBURST, BUT HAS A
SIMILAR RESULT. YOU "DEAL"
WITH THE ISSUE QUICKLY, BUT
THEN ESCAPE. YOU HIDE.

WHAT'S THE POINT?

That said, let's go back to the main idea of this chapter:

> *Emotions are part of who we are. If we don't find a healthy way to express them, our feelings "come out" in unhealthy ways.*

Over the next few pages we're going to take a short trip- a trek that will encourage, equip, and empower us to recognize the emotions that are filling "our balloon." Rather than reacting in unhealthy ways, we'll be able to:

- Recognize those emotions.

- Realize the truth of what they're saying (and not saying).

- Respond in a healthy way that honors us and the people around us.

That said, let's go to the next page and explore a foundational concept- the truth that we'll never be healthier than our emotional wholeness.

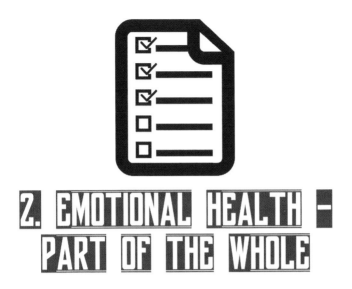

2. EMOTIONAL HEALTH – PART OF THE WHOLE

MAIN IDEA= EMOTIONAL HEALTH IS A VITAL COMPONENT OF TOTAL HEALTH- YET IT'S ONE THAT WE OFTEN OVERLOOK. AND, THE REALITY IS THAT YOU WON'T BE HEALTHY WITHOUT EMOTIONAL WHOLENESS.

About two years ago I found myself in a six-month long funk. Enacting option #3 from the previous chapter, I blew off a bit of steam and then went numb. I entered a long season of depression. It was Spring 2017.

During that time, I read Peter Scazzero's book *Emotionally Healthy Spirituality*.

Then I double-dipped. I downloaded his material on Audible, so I could review it as I ran, drove, and performed routine chores around the house. I felt I needed an ongoing refresher on the contents. I had no idea how powerful and useful his insights would prove to me.

In the book, Scazzero reminds us, first of all, that we are multifaceted people- each of us having various components:

1. Physical

2. Spiritual

3. Intellectual

4. Social / relational

5. Emotional

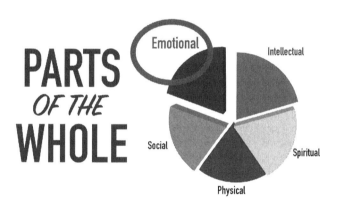

Most of us readily identify with four of these areas- the first four. However, Scazzero observes that many people walk through life with an under-developed emotional center. He recalls precisely what many of us could likely say about ourselves:

> I had been taught the way to approach life was through fact, and feelings, in that order... [feelings were] dangerous and needed to be suppressed.[3]

---

[3] This quote comes from *Emotionally Healthy Spirituality*.

Whereas we don't need to make permanent decisions based on temporary feelings we need to acknowledge our emotions were given to us by God. Remember what we saw in the first chapter? **If you don't proactively deal with your emotions, at some point they build up and you end up reacting in one of the three unhealthy ways.**

WHAT PULLS YOU?

Scazzero's observation resonated with me...

I remember a Gospel tract I saw when I was a kid. Gospel tracts are small brochures designed to tell people about Jesus.[4] An entire page in the back of the religious pamphlet was designed to explain how we might not always feel "saved."

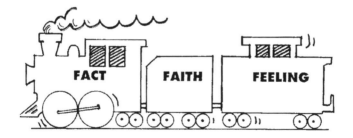

The writer used a train to illustrate the point, making the analogy simple:

---

[4] I grew up Southern Baptist. These pamphlets were a way of life.

- **Facts are the engine.** They pull the train (and us) where we need to go.

- **Faith is the coal car, the fuel**. Faith provides life and "fire" to the facts.

Both of these are needed. Without facts the train won't have any horsepower. Without faith that engine will never catch spark and do what it's designed to do.

There's another component to the train, though, *the caboose*. Look at the label on the picture. Yes, the tract suggested feelings are the final part of the train.

"The train will run with or without the caboose," the author explained.

Think about it. That's a true statement. After all, what *is* the purpose of the caboose- besides signifying you've reached the end of the train? I see trains coasting through our neighborhood without one almost daily.

But in life…

Are feelings *actually unnecessary*? Are our emotions *unneeded*?

Now, I don't know that the author of the brochure was making *that* argument. (And in the previous chapter we saw that your emotions eventually do reveal themselves- even if they do so in unhealthy ways). But, **I do believe that's where we've taken things: *we need the facts; we need faith; we can take or leave the feelings.***

But if we leave feelings out of the equation our emotions become under-developed. And that can be tricky.

Let me convey it like Scazzero does…

Remember the five areas I listed a few pages ago? Let's look at the first four…

1. **Physical.** Scazzero observes that if we see someone with a physical handicap we make concessions for them. We go out of our way to assist the man sitting in the wheelchair or the woman walking with a cane. We help people wearing casts and braces and other signifiers that their body is in repair.

2. **Spiritual.** In church and religious circles we learn to do the same with people who struggle spiritually. We answer their questions, we point them to truth, and we walk with them through their struggle. Their "issues," too, are generally obvious. They broadcast their struggle as they express doubts and voice concerns.

3. **Intellectual.** Scazzero reminds us that we usually notice people who have intellectual struggles. We assist them, too. Whether it's Alzheimer's disease, Tourette syndrome, or even a learning disability, we embrace people with mental challenges and help meet their needs.

4. **Social / relational.** Scazzero notes that we make concessions for people who may be socially or relationally awkward. We understand that some people are just… well… odd. We offer them the benefit of the doubt- and loads of grace.

Now, two of the primary reasons we're able to extend such grace in the four scenarios above is because…

1. **The issue is obvious**- be it a physical, intellectual, spiritual, or relational "defect." The person with the issue and others around them both notice what's happening. *And,*

2. **The issue is owned**. The person with the issue generally knows they have some sort of impediment standing between them and optimal health.

MOST ISSUES...

OBVIOUS = CAN'T HIDE THEM
OWNED = ADMIT HAVING THEM

BUT EMOTIONAL DYSFUNCTION...

The problem with emotional unhealth is that, unlike these other areas, it often goes unseen- particularly when spirituality is present. In fact, Scazzero argues that people with a regular religious routine may actually go more unnoticed when they're emotionally unhealthy.

Furthermore, the issue may be unnoticeable to the person as well as to those around them… for a while. In time, bystanders recognize the flaw, as they begin to feel the control of the "drama" the person brings with them to virtually every situation in which they're involved.

However, the perpetrator may not be aware of how they're perceived! Or, if they're truly emotionally unhealthy, they may actually think everyone else has an issue... and that they have some sort of "enlightenment."

Spirituality often masks emotional dysfunction- even unintentionally. If you look good spiritually, people assume you're fine emotionally. If you know how to pray, if you raise your hands while you sing in church, if you talk about your relationship with God easily... people just assume you're emotionally healthy.

In fact, you may actually fool yourself! You may find yourself claiming "direct revelation" or "supernatural insight" that the "spirit" gives you- even revelation that contradicts things clearly written in Scripture.[5]

(You might not only fool yourself into thinking you're healthy; you might actually be one of the most unhealthy people of all!)

In other words, going back to the two points above-

1. **Obvious.** Emotional issues might not be obvious.

2. **Owned.** The person with the issue may not be aware they have an issue!

For years- no, decades- this is where I was. I left a wake of hurt and pain behind me. This wasn't due to the religious things I taught. Rather, it was connected to the way I handled myself emotionally.

---

[5] Paul was aware of this happening even during his times. He wrote, "But even if we or an angel from heaven should preach a gospel other than the one we preached to you, let them be under God's curse" (Galatians 1:8 NIV). Later, Peter wrote, "knowing this first of all, that no prophecy of Scripture comes from someone's own interpretation" (2 Peter 1:20). In other words, we don't get to redefine truth to suit our emotional dysfunction. More about this in chapter 3.

"The stuff you taught when you were working at the church was right on," a previous co-staff member recently told me, as we reconnected after 7-plus years of total silence. "There was something about how you were doing things, though…"

We were sitting in a coffee shop. As I listened to his words, all spoken to me in love, I thought back through my story…

The lying, the dishonesty, the manipulation… the bullying, the blaming, and the finding my identity and worth in what I did as opposed to who I am… Those are all emotionally-based issues. **I've seen that my total health, including my spiritual vitality, will never be higher than my emotional wholeness.**

"I'm sorry," he said. "I loved you, but I didn't love you enough to say, 'Hey! Let's look at these things here!'"

I had some strong areas for sure. But I also had a weak area. One we over-looked. And it caused me to crash.

Remember what I mentioned in the intro? **Emotions are a big deal but we give them very little attention…**

Look at it this way: a 20-link chain with 19 links can carry 1,500 pounds and one link that can hold only 15 pounds will never lift more than 15 pounds. Regardless of how powerful the other 19 are, they're held back by the weak link. That's easy to understand, right?

Well, in the same way a chain will never prove stronger than its weakest link, well…. neither will we. Think about it with me…

- If you're mentally strong and have great ideas that will change the world, you'll never be able to do it unless you're healthy. It's hard to be a world-changer when you're sick in the bed.

- If you're spiritually stout but can't relate to others... you'll have a difficult time conveying the deep truths the Lord delivers to you while you're in your prayer closet.

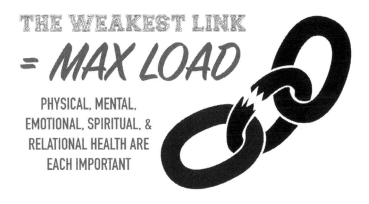

THE WEAKEST LINK = MAX LOAD

PHYSICAL, MENTAL, EMOTIONAL, SPIRITUAL, & RELATIONAL HEALTH ARE EACH IMPORTANT

Emotional dysfunction is an easy trap to fall into, because we don't value emotional well-being in the same way we value physical health, intellectual wholeness, spiritual growth, and social relate-ability. Now, I don't know that the author of the brochure with the train pic was making the argument that we don't *need* our emotions. But, that's where we've taken things. We need the facts; we need faith; we can take or leave the feelings.

GROWING EMOTIONAL INTELLIGENCE

This past year I picked up the book *Emotional Intelligence 2.0*. Yes, I have the actual book *and* I downloaded it via Audible, as well!

2. EMOTIONAL HEALTH = PART OF THE WHOLE

Here's a key statement from the book:

> *Emotional Intelligence is your ability to recognize and understand emotions in yourself and others, and your ability to use this awareness to manage your behavior and relationships.*[6]

I read some of the statements to a group of several hundred men at Advance 10.0 this past Fall in Minnesota.[7] Some of them were spellbound by the data, with findings that suggest Emotional Quotient (EQ) is a greater indicator of future success than Intelligence Quotient (IQ). For instance-

- People with the highest IQ levels out-perform those with average IQ scores *only* 20% of the time.[8]

- Average IQ people out-perform high IQ people 70% of the time![9]

This one factor proves incredibly interesting. We typically think the *greatest* predictor of future success is IQ. After all, that seems to be what most schools evaluate for admissions. It's certainly what schools "grade" as we take our classes. And, when we look back at "how we did" while we were in school, IQ-related information-regurgitation is how we assess ourselves.

But, when the data is reviewed, the numbers are profound. We see that our Emotional Quotient seems to be a more important number. Notice-

- 90% of high performers have high EQ

---

[6] *Emotional Intelligence 2.0*, Travis Bradberry & Jean Graves, Kindle Version, location 334.

[7] Go to www.EatSleepAdvance.com for more info.

[8] *Emotional Intelligence 2.0*, Travis Bradberry & Jean Graves, Kindle Version, location 257.

[9] *Emotional Intelligence 2.0*, Travis Bradberry & Jean Graves, Kindle Version, location 257.

- 20% of low performers have high EQ[10]

People with high EQ make more money- an average of $29,000 more per year- than people with low EQ. In fact, every point on the test in Emotional Intelligence 2.0 accounted for a $1,300 uptick in annual salary- across all career fields.[11]

This isn't just "field specific," either. Emotional Quotient accounts for 58% performance in *all types of jobs*...

> It's the single biggest predictor of performance in the workplace and the strongest driver of leadership and personal excellence.[12]

If you- like me- feel like you've got a long way to go emotionally, don't despair. Whereas IQ (our ability to assimilate new information and learn) is a relatively static and unchanging number, EQ- like your physical strength and stamina- can actually grow!

Or, to say it another way, ""EQ is a flexible skill that can be learned."[13]

That means this: we can all work on- *and develop*- the area that is the greatest indicator of success in the future.

In other words, we'll never be stronger than the weakest "part" of our whole person. Yet, emotions are clearly an area where we can grow!

---

[10] Stats found in *Emotional Intelligence 2.0*, Travis Bradberry & Jean Graves, Kindle Version, location 366.

[11] *Emotional Intelligence 2.0*, Travis Bradberry & Jean Graves, Kindle Version, location 366.

[12] *Emotional Intelligence 2.0*, Travis Bradberry & Jean Graves, Kindle Version, location 358.

[13] *Emotional Intelligence 2.0*, Travis Bradberry & Jean Graves, Kindle Version, location 334.

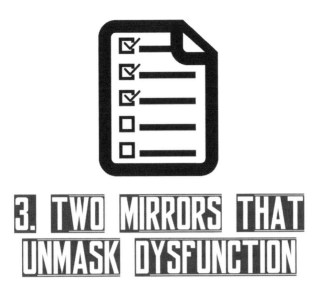

3. TWO MIRRORS THAT UNMASK DYSFUNCTION

MAIN IDEA= SPIRITUALITY OFTEN MASKS EMOTIONAL DYSFUNCTION. TWO THINGS TRANSFORM US INTO WHO WE'RE DESIGNED TO BE, THOUGH, MAKING US SPIRITUALLY HEALTHY & EMOTIONALLY WHOLE!

A few pages ago I mentioned that spiritual health often masks emotional dysfunction. If you look good spiritually, people assume you're emotionally whole. You might not be. In fact, you might be outright destructive. Furthermore, you may even fool yourself!

Here's one of the reasons why: spiritual things *look* emotional. And, we've been taught that emotional experiences (i.e.,. goosebumps in church) are signs of spirituality- even though football games, birthday gifts, and songs on the radio can elicit the exact same emotional response.

In other words, **emotional ≠ spiritual anymore than non-emotional ≠ non-spiritual**. The two are mutually exclusive.

Think about it…

- *How many emotionally unstable people have argued against something by taking the spiritual high ground- even though they were wrong?* (It's impossible to have a healthy conversation with someone who plays the trump card of "God told me," isn't it?)

- *How many times have you seen someone throw themselves into volunteerism, humanitarian causes, and- yes- even ministry in order to meet their own (often unseen) emotional needs?* (Been there, done it, have the t-shirt and scars to prove it.)

- *How often have you seen people in positions of spiritual leadership use the Bible like a barrage of bullets, resorting to spiritual manipulation to get their way, leaving a trail of destruction behind them?* (Again, I'm speaking to the man in the mirror on this one.)

Because of scenarios like the three I just mentioned, a lot of people speak against "religion."

Or they say things like, "I like Jesus, but not religion."

And, "I love God but I hate theology."

I understand.

Religion *CAN BE* reduced to rules and legalism and… *control*. And theology *CAN BE* a construct we use to argue for that control.

But the word *theology* means "what we know and believe about God."

And the word *religion* means "reconnect."

The reality is that God came near to reconnect us to Himself *AND* to reconnect us to each other (in a healthy way) *AND* to reconnect us to our true selves. In other words, *theology* and *religion* are powerful words when used in the right way!

Religion
Re-ligio
RE-CONNECT

THE SOLUTION = TO RE-CONNECT

The Scripture teaches us that two things transform us into the image of Christ. Not seventy. Not twelve. Not five. *Two…*

These *both* have *everything* to do with reconnecting us to the Father and reconnecting us to each other. Let's take a deep dive into them.

First, looking at Christ transforms us into His image.

There's a now-famous guy Jesus meets early in His ministry. True to form, Jesus completely changes this man's name, restoring his fractured identity and reconnecting him to who he really is.

Here's the snip from John 1:42 where we see it happen (ESV):

> Jesus looked at him and said, "You are Simon the son of John. You shall be called Cephas" (which means Peter).

That's it. It's the first time Jesus encounters the fisherman, according to John. And, it seems *completely* insignificant until you get more info.

The name Simon literally means "reed, twig, shifting sand." If this man behaves in any way related to what he's been named by his parents, it means that he is:

- *Undependable*- he might change from one moment to the next

- *Unreliable*- he will likely say he's going to do one thing but then do the exact opposite

- *Unstable*- his emotions might throw him off balance

Turns out, the name Jesus gives him is the *exact opposite* of his given name. Jesus calls him *Peter*, that is "rock." Whereas you can't build anything on quicksand, rock is stable and steady. It's what you desperately *want*.

Remember, Jesus gives Peter this new name *the first time He meets him*. He literally speaks destiny into him when he does.

The problem is that, well... Peter is *everything but a rock* for the next several pages of Scripture. And it's not like he's "all bad." Rather he's shifty- like sand. He bends- like a twig. He sinks after trying to walk on water (Matthew 8:25). He rebukes Jesus for stating He's going to the Cross (Matthew 16:22). He falls asleep when Jesus asks him to pray for Him in the Garden of Gethsemane (Mark 14:37f.). He denies Jesus three times, even cursing that he doesn't even know Him (Matthew 26:69f.). Then, even after seeing the empty tomb, he abandons being a disciple and goes back his previous job of fishing (John 21:3f.).

Later, Peter turns things around. He becomes the rock Jesus says he is. He takes charge of the disciples and helps them elect a new leader to replace Judas (Acts 1:15). He preaches at Pentecost and 3,000 people come to faith (Acts 2:14f.). He heals a lame beggar with a word, without even praying (Acts 3:6). He's arrested for preaching, then preaches during his trial (Acts 4:8,19). He walks in such power that even his shadow heals people (Acts 5:15). He even raises the dead (Acts 9:40-41).

So what do we make of this?

Well, **we know that Jesus came to show us what the Father is like.** That's why He tells us things like:

- "Whoever has seen me has seen the Father" (John 14:9).

- "The words I speak aren't just mine- they're the Father's words (John 14:24).

- "I only do what I see the Father doing" (John 5:19).

In other words, **Jesus reveals what God is like.** He's the exact representation of God (Colossians 1:15, Hebrews 1:3), and the fullness of the deity literally dwells in Him (Colossians 2:9).

That is...

- **Jesus introduces us to the Father.** That is, He shows us who God really is. (Hence, a recovery of powerful, hope-filled words like *religion* and *theology*.)

For our purposes on this topic, though, here's what I *really* want you to see...

- **Jesus also introduces us to ourselves.** *He shows us who we really are.*

Think about that *first* exchange between Peter and Jesus. Here's what actually happened:

"Hey, Simon, let me tell you who I am. My name is Jesus… I'm here to show you what the Father is really like."

Then, before Peter can grasp what that actually means, Jesus continues. "By the way, I'm here to show you who you really are, too. And, with that, let's just start right here… you're *not* the wavering, waffling guy that you seem to be… you're not your past, no matter how present that past seems to be… I've designed you for greatness. **And when you look at me, you're going to not only see who the Father is, you're going to see who you are, too."**

Sounds strange, doesn't it?

Paul penned it like this (2 Corinthians 3:18 NKJV):

> *…we all, with unveiled face,* **beholding as in a mirror** *the glory of the Lord, are being* **transformed into the same image** *from glory to glory, just as by the Spirit of the Lord.*

Did you catch it? Paul said that looking at Jesus is *just like looking at yourself in a mirror.* And, the more we look at the image of Jesus, the more we're transformed into that likeness, the more it seems that we're looking into a mirror.

John (one of the disciples who spent a lot of time with Peter) wrote it like this: "We will have confidence in the day of judgment, because **in this world we are like Him**" (1 John 4:17).

I love what John says- a lot of people are afraid of approaching God because of their sin issues. Because they've waffled like Simon. They've had some great moments and some "nonsense" moments.

Yet, even in that, John says there's no fear of judgment, that I'm not "like that," *because I'm like Jesus.*

And Paul says **we're so much like Jesus that when we look at Jesus it's like we're seeing our own reflection in the mirror.**

I know. Mind-blown. Right?

FORGETTING WHAT'S IN THE MIRROR

The trouble is that **we continue looking everywhere else to find something that we already have.**

The truth is that we actually *become* the extreme version of whatever we focus on…

- *Focus on money* = we become greedy

- *Focus on sex* = we become lustful

- *Focus on rest* = we become lazy

- *Focus on work* = we become overbearing and start striving and "hustling" for the things that are freely ours

Now, each of these things- money, sex, rest, and work- are incredible gifts. But, they're not ours to "behold." They're ours to *receive* and to *enjoy.*

Think about how many of our emotional issues come from chasing these things!

James, Jesus' little brother, says not to fall for that trap. He writes,

> *For if anyone is a hearer of the word and not a doer, he is* **like a man observing his natural face in a mirror; for he observes himself, goes away, and immediately forgets what kind of man he was** *(James 1:23-24 NKJV).*

Let me ask you this: *I bet if I showed you a picture of yourself you would recognize your own face, wouldn't you?*

How so? Because you've seen yourself in a mirror. *You know what you actually look like.*

(Yeah, *even little kids* recognize themselves in family pictures or on the camera reel of your smartphone!)

There's no way you'd be confused *about you*, correct?

Yet James says this is *exactly* what we're prone to do. Spiritually, anyway.

He says it's exactly the same. **In the same way that we don't forget who we are physically, we shouldn't forget who we are in Christ**- as new creations, as His image bearers, as people for whom He's called forth greatness.

It means we don't get "tripped up" over our mess-ups. Like Peter, we'll have episodes in which the evidence seems to suggest that we're not who Jesus says we are. In time, though, Jesus is right- 100% of the time.

Again, **the first thing that transforms us into the image of Christ… the thing that reconnects us to our Heavenly Father is beholding Jesus Himself**. That leads us to the second thing that reconnects us…

THE SECOND TRANSFORMATIONAL TOOL

Second, looking at others transforms us into (their and) His image.

In fact, Solomon says it clearly:

> *As iron sharpens iron, so the countenance of one man sharpens another (Proverbs 27:17).*

A *countenance* is "face." That is, **the face of others- up close and personal- has the power to change us.**

One author said it well: "The person you are in five years is the sum total of the books you read and the five people with whom you spend the most time."

When I was in high school a youth minister of mine repeatedly reminded us: "Show me your friends, and I'll show you your future."

Two things transform us into who we're designed to be

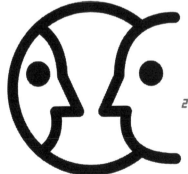

1. THE IMAGE OF CHRIST
2 CORINTHIANS 3:18

2. THE COUNTENANCE OF OTHERS
PROVERBS 27:17

FIND THEM NOW

One of the most powerful things you can do for your overall health is to find a group of people who will journey with you. Now, I don't mean a group of "fans" (one-way relationships with people who look up to you and endorse everything you do) or "acquaintances" (surface level relationships that don't have the relational weight to carry tough conversations) but- rather- *truly deep friendships*. The kind the Bible describes. The ones who sharpen you (Proverbs 27:17). The ones who can tell you what you don't want to hear that you desperately need to hear (Proverbs 27:6).

That last one is important.

I meet people all the time who *suggest* they have a group of accountability partners who walk with them- people who tell them what they *need* to hear. Turns out, though, they often *don't*. Rather, they have a group of acquaintance-friends who will tell them what they *want* to hear, but won't challenge them when they need it the most.

Those "accountability" partners confess, "Yes, I love _____, and we're friends, but our relationship won't carry the weight of me telling them _____ " (insert the name of some major issue where the person needs emotional correction).

Often, they say the friend will cut them off emotionally or relationally... or argue back against them.

In other word, their emotional dysfunction surfaces!

That's not a true transformational support system. A support system should be designed to uphold us when we're crashing- *even when we don't know we're crashing*. In fact, that's when we most need it, right!?

That means it's important to walk closely with people who know you well and have the right to speak into your life. Often, that entails actually communicating to them that you sincerely want them to challenge you, to call forth the greatness that's in you- even if it means correcting you and telling you hard truths.

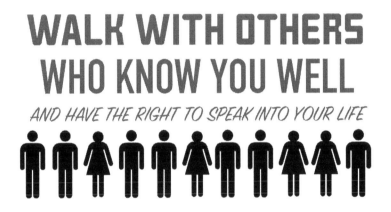

WALK WITH OTHERS
WHO KNOW YOU WELL
AND HAVE THE RIGHT TO SPEAK INTO YOUR LIFE

BLIND SPOTS - WE ALL HAVE THEM

The reality is that we all have blind spots. I used to think I didn't have any. **By their very definition, blind spots are hidden places you can't see.** They're *obvious* to everyone else- particularly to the people closest to you. But, they're invisible to you even as they sit in plain site.

BLIND SPOTS

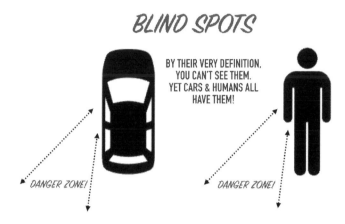

BY THEIR VERY DEFINITION,
YOU CAN'T SEE THEM.
YET CARS & HUMANS ALL
HAVE THEM!

DANGER ZONE!   *DANGER ZONE!*

Furthermore- and this is the glory of it- **our blind spots might hide hidden dangers or they may hide hidden beauties we need to see**. In other words, don't think of accountability in the negative sense only- as a group of people telling us what *not* to do... think of accountability as a group of people empowering us to be all that we can be.

That is, our support system may say, "Hey, watch out- you're not seeing this right."

Or, they might say, "Look, there's something great about you here that you need to see. Let me remind you of it..."

This means that we don't get side-swiped when others don't live up to who they really are, either- any more than Jesus did when Peter continued failing. We continue, like Christ, calling forth the image in the mirror. That means that, sometimes, we even see that image in them before they do, right?

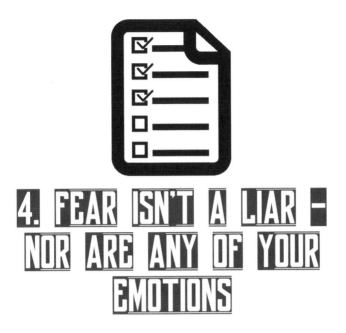

4. FEAR ISN'T A LIAR – NOR ARE ANY OF YOUR EMOTIONS

MAIN IDEA= THERE AREN'T BAD EMOTIONS AND GOOD EMOTIONS. JUST HEALTHY AND UNHEALTHY EXPRESSIONS OF ALL OF THEM.

I was listening to the radio the other day and heard the mantra, "Fear is a liar…"

Then someone posted a meme on Instagram that said the same thing.

Though it *sounds* true, and though I understand the sentiment behind this "bumper sticker-ism," fear isn't a liar. Rather, fear is a valid emotion, an expression of something happening deep inside (often because of some external circumstance) that our heart seeks to communicate to us.

If you're about to step off the edge of a cliff, fear is healthy. Fear might save you from walking down a dark alley, keep you from engaging in a verbal barrage with a bully, or trying to cross a railroad track when there's an oncoming train. You get the idea.

No, we don't want to be controlled by fear, but we do want to hear what our hearts are saying.

That leads me to this…

We're often afraid to talk about- or even feel- the "bad" emotions. We've been told that *fear* and *anger* and some of the other emotions aren't healthy. Hence the "bumper sticker-isms," memes, and pithy one-liners.

Let me offer a different perspective: **There aren't bad emotions and good emotions. Just healthy and unhealthy expressions of all of them**. Many of us are taught- from a young age- to be afraid of the "bad" emotions. But, we shouldn't be.

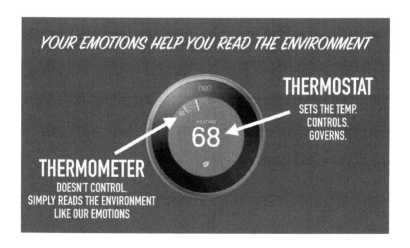

Make note: a thermostat *sets* the temperature in the environment; a thermometer simply tells you what the temperature is. **Once we learn the emotions are thermometers- telling us the temperature of the world around us rather than controlling that temperature- we're better suited to deal with reality and navigate our way through life.**

You see, this enables us to "read" the environment, sense what's happening, and then adjust the climate appropriately.

(We'll come back to this concept when we review the Emotional Wholeness Checklist in chapter 5 and discuss how to work through its 3-step process in any situation.)

HEART WORK

Last year I taught an emotional health workshop at the church in Prattville, Alabama. During that time, I shared the following graphic with the group. They were the first group to every see it.

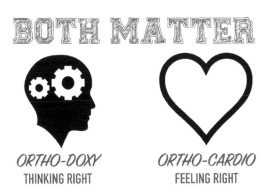

BOTH MATTER

ORTHO-DOXY
THINKING RIGHT

ORTHO-CARDIO
FEELING RIGHT

I created it because I've realized that a big part of our "inside work" is our emotional health, not just the spiritual truths we intellectually profess. That is, both are important- right thinking and right feeling. Again, we're back to that "chain is only as strong as the weakest link" thing.

I've shared the image a few times since then, and it always catches some people off-guard. Honestly, before my journey of healing it would have shaken me, too.

But let me show you something- a truth so obvious I missed it until recently.

See if you can complete the following sentence.

The Bible tells us, "God is _____."

Yeah, you probably nailed it. A lot of people do...

"God is *love*" (1 John 4:8).

We're so familiar with the phrase that we forget *love* **is both a commitment of unconditional covenant** *and* **love is an emotion.** God, though committed to us, is emotional, too. He doesn't just accept us because He's chosen to commit Himself to us; He's *passionate* about us. That is, there's an emotional component to how He relates to us.

THE GOOD, THE BAD, THE UGLY

In the previous chapter I mentioned that Jesus shows us what we're like and He shows us what the Father is like. Remember that...

Throughout the New Testament we read truths like-

- Jesus wept multiple times, including at Lazarus' tomb (John 11:35) and even over the city of Jerusalem itself (see Luke 13:35, 19:41).

- Jesus became angry on several occasions. He overturned the money changers' tables in the temple, after taking the time to make a whip to loosen the sacrificial animals (John 2:15, Matthew 21:12). He expressed His indignation when the disciples brushed the little children way from Him (Mark 10:14).

- Jesus was distressed with the Pharisees (Mark 3:5).

- Jesus was moved with compassion (Mark 6:34).

- Jesus was full of joy through the Holy Spirit (Luke 10:21).

- Jesus was sorrowful and troubled (Matthew 26:37-38).

- Jesus lingers even now, because the Lord is patient (2 Peter 3:9).

We see all of the emotions- the "good" side and "bad" side- in the life of Jesus.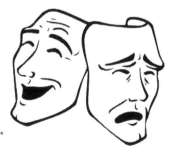

In God (Jesus is God) we see the full range of emotions- even the ones we typically consider to be "bad" or "taboo" ones- expressed in a healthy way.

Now, think about this (and connect it to what we learned in the previous chapter about being transformed into His likeness!)-

- Since we're created in His image, *and...*

- Since we're being transformed into His image (as we behold Him as well as walk with others who are being awakened to that same image)...

- We don't have to be afraid of any of these emotions.

Leif Heitland, a Bible teacher, locked-on to this notion of God's feelings. He writes,

> *I often ask God to share His emotions with me because I know He is an emotional God- full of compassion, joy, and many other feelings.* [14]

Sometimes these feelings are "negative." We become broken for other people, as we see them dealing with pain.

There aren't GOOD emotions & BAD emotions.

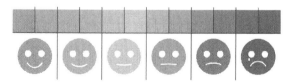

---

[14] Leif Heitland, *Called to Reign*, page 125.

Sometimes we become broken for ourselves. I can't tell you how many times I've broken down and cried as I've worked my way through my story- as I've seen the hurt done to me, as I've sensed the pain I've inflicted on my wife and family, as I've realized how much I have exposed my loved ones to spiritual and real danger.

There aren't "bad" emotions, in other words. Our emotions communicate the temperature of our soul to us. And, again, since we're created in God's image, we should expect to experience the same emotions Jesus did.

TIME TO BECOME SELF-AWARE

Solomon tells us, "There is a time to weep and a time to laugh... a time to mourn and a time to dance" (Ecclesiastes 3:4). Notice *both extremes* of the emotional scale are present.

Paul acknowledged that we grieve, but "we do not grieve as those who have no hope" (1 Thessalonians 4:13). That is, the emotion is present- even if we express it in a different way than others who lack hope.

Grasp that final sentence. It's important. **Feeling an emotion doesn't mean we *must* express it in an unhealthy way.** Remember, the emotion doesn't set the temperature and control the environment (like a thermostat); it simply reads the climate and communicates what's happening (like a thermometer). **Feeling the raw, unfiltered emotion simply means... well... we're not afraid to allow ourselves to sense what's actually happening in our heart.**

I used to believe emotions could be dangerous- that we could be deceived or led astray by them. And that we should *never* rely on our feelings. Or, to say it another way (like we referenced earlier in the book), "You shouldn't let the caboose pull the train."

Maybe there's some accuracy to that. But the truth is that-

- Faith can lead us astray, too, *if that faith rests on the wrong thing.*

- Facts- *if they're the wrong facts-* can derail us too.

(This is one of the huge reasons I advocate walking in close relationship with others- people to whom you grant authority to challenge you and uphold you at the same time. They can help you explore your emotions, as well as insure you're listening to what they say without making poor decisions based on them.)

For years I wanted to run from emotions rather than running towards them. It seemed safer, easier. Yet the way towards health and healing is actually to move straight into the emotions rather than trying to navigate around them.

To do this ,though, you must grow in self-awareness. The authors of *Emotional Intelligence 2.0* say that "To be self aware is to know yourself as you really are."

Part of "knowing yourself" is being able to read what your heart is saying. The stats say that only 36% of the people tested- 1/3- can identify their own feelings as they happen.[15]

One of the reasons we have trouble identifying our emotions, I think, is because we're still afraid to admit it when we sense the "bad" ones. Maybe a perspective from how our physical bodies work will help…

---

[15] And, "Facing the truth about who you are can at times be unsettling. Getting in touch with your emotions and tendencies takes honesty and courage" *Emotional Intelligence 2.0*, Travis Bradberry & Jean Graves, Kindle Version, location 769).

The emotion isn't "Good" or "Bad." It's what we do with it...

PAIN IS [KINDA] YOUR FRIEND

Pain isn't the enemy emotionally anymore than it is physically. Most of us do our best to *avoid* emotional pain. We bury it. We explain it away.

Think about the need for physical pain, though...

A few years ago, our son Judah broke his arm. He tripped on the playground, landed awkwardly as he tried to catch himself, and his forearm snapped in half. Every kid and teacher on the playground actually *heard* it.

The break was so complete that he had to hold the "broken off" part of his arm in place lest it just dangle. The physical wound was *obvious*. Physical defects and wounds are usually *obvious* and *owned* by the person; emotional ones are not. It makes it even more difficult to navigate this when we avoid the tough emotions.

About a year later our daughter Mini fell from the zip line in our backyard.[16] She was shaken up a bit, so we took her inside and let her take a warm bath.

---

16 That's my nickname for Miriam.

An hour or two after the fall, she complained of pain in her wrist. It looked fine (no dangling loose like Judah's left arm), but the sting persisted. We took her to the emergency room and learned she had a small sprain. We discovered this *because* of the pain. Or, to say it another way, *if she didn't experience the pain we wouldn't have known about the sprain.*

In the same way that physical pain alerts us to the reality that something isn't quite right in our body, emotional pain reveals the truth about our soul. Emotional wounds tell us that something's not quite right.

As Brennan Manning writes,

> Whether positive or negative, feelings put us in touch with our true selves. They are neither good nor bad. *[Emotions] are simply the truth of what is going on within us*.[17]

Another author reminds us,

> The Hebrew & Greek words for heart are used almost 1,000 times in Scripture, making it the most anthropological term in the Bible. **Your heart is such a big deal to God that He writes about it more than anything else- more than sin, more than works, more than obedience, even more than love**. And according to God, the heart designed actually determines the course of your life.[18]

The truth is that the heart is intimately connected to all of life.

- The words we say are birthed in our hearts (Proverbs 10:11, Matthew 12:34, Luke 6:45).

---

[17] Brennan Manning, *Abba's Child*, Kindle version- location 1348.

[18] Christa Black Gifford, *Heart Made Whole*, Kindle version- location 567.

- Our heart reveals the motives others may not see in our actions (Proverbs 24:12).

- The things we do- our actions- originate in the heart (Mark 7:21).

Everything we do is an overflow of the heart inside of us.

The Scripture shows me that God can be found in our emotions. And that seeking the Kingdom often involves not simply doing things out in the world but also in doing the tough, deep work of the soul. That means exploring what's happening inside- and uncovering why- and then having a way to respond when things occur. And that leads us to the Emotional Wholeness Checklist.

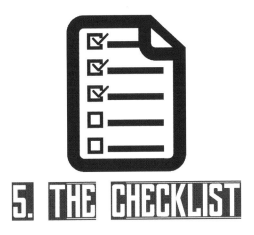

5. THE CHECKLIST

MAIN IDEA= WE AREN'T REQUIRED TO REACT WHEN WE RECOGNIZE AN EMOTIONAL FEELING. RATHER, WE CAN STEP BACK AND "READ" WHAT OUR HEART IS SAYING. THEN, WE CAN RESPOND IN A HEALTHY MANNER.

Most of us don't have trouble expressing ourselves when things are going well. We smile. We laugh. We clap. We feel and exhibit joy.

The trouble comes when things don't go like we planned, right? When we face the "struggle bus" or something of the like…

One of the authors of the Testament, James, says to "Count it all joy *when you endure trials*" (James 1:2).

You read that correctly. He says to *express* a happy emotion when you face a tough circumstance.

Now, his statement presumes both of the following:

- **First, we can correctly feel the weight of a tough circumstance *without* hiding our hearts from it.** That is, we're not afraid of the "bad" emotions. We correctly label what we're facing as a "trial" (or whatever it happens to be).

- **Second, we can control our response to the situation and actually feel joy- despite that circumstance.** That is, we allow our emotions to function like thermometers (reading the climate)- not thermostats (setting the climate). We have the capacity to respond to unhealthy situations in healthy ways.

In other words, James contends that **even when we can't control the externals, we can take charge of what happens inside of us**.

Sounds like a tall order. In fact, it sounds *almost impossible*.

James promises something to those who endure the dark night. In James 1:3-4, he says to consider it joy-

> because you know that the testing of your faith produces perseverance. Let perseverance finish its work so that you may be mature and complete, not lacking anything.

That is, tough situations take us to the "end" of ourselves, to a place where we can no longer rely on our personal resources. At that point, the Spirit produces something *new* and *substantial* inside us- something beautiful and strong that can't be acquired from any other place.

When tough scenarios used to arise, I acted quickly- and immaturely. Quickly. Impulsively. I *reacted* instead of pausing to reflect and read what was happening. I acted *emotionally*- in the bad sense of the word. I let my emotions become the thermostat (setting the environment) rather than serve as a thermometer (communicating to me what was happening).

James says to step back.

Focus.

Endure the struggle.

Let God do His perfect work in you because that will pour forth, overflowing out of you into your situation.

Because I was unwilling to deal with the difficult emotions (embracing healthy limitations about what I could achieve, feeling like a failure if something didn't work out, accepting rejection if people stepped away from me for failing), I walked in deception.

The tricky thing about deception is that, by the very definition of being deceived (tricked, led astray, manipulated) you don't realize what's happening in the moment. You rationalize your position.

No one (self-included) has every said, "Hmmm... I'm being deceived right now."

We fool ourselves. That's what it means to be deceived.

(Hence the need to have a small group of truth-tellers whom we regularly invite into our lives, people who can see those blind spots and speak freely to us about them.)

When we walk in deception, choosing to ignore the reality of what's happening around us and to us, we can no longer see who we really are as opposed to who we're trying to be. We move into "image-management" rather than "image-transformation." The image in the mirror becomes fuzzy, faded… a distant memory.

The solution?

Go back. Embrace the dark night. Do the tough work. **Cease the image management and embrace the mess.** That's where you find healing.

THE AMAZING WORK...

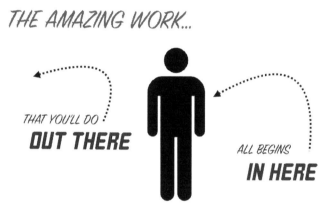

THAT YOU'LL DO
OUT THERE

ALL BEGINS
IN HERE

Peter Scazzero says that the verse from James "carries with it the notion of God importing or infusing something of His character into us through the process of difficulties and severe trials."[19] **In those rough patches that God imparts something to us that's only available to be received from the tough places.**

Think about it-

---

[19] From *Emotionally Healthy Spirituality.*

- David ran for his life for 13 years. Yet, afterwards, he was able to lead people with such grace and kindness, living with the heart of the Father and overlooking insults (see 2 Samuel 16:5).

- Job endured his dark night and later confessed, "I had heard of God before, but now I've seen Him face-to-face" (Job 42:5). He, then, was able to bless his friends, the very ones who mocked him and caused additional pain throughout his journey (Job 42:10).

- Joseph, the boy who wore the multi-colored robe, knew his destiny from the beginning. But he walked in arrogance. Others rejected him. After enduring the dungeon, he rose to prominence. He rescued two nations, Egypt and Israel, after reaching a state of emotional health that empowered him to honor his betrayers from both people groups (see Genesis 37:8f.).

The "outside" fruit we see in each of these lives was a result of the great work that happened on the inside. Like James says, God worked something in them as they travailed through the mess.

WORTH THE WORK

Dealing with emotions is tough work. I've learned- *no, I'm learning*- it's worth the journey, though. **It never seems like it during the "patient endurance" phase. However, there are things I've acquired in my soul which I'm convinced weren't available to be any other way**.

Often, just when I'm ready to move forward with life, and get on with the "good stuff," for things to be "easy," my Father imparts even more to me, showing that it's good for me- though trying- to journey through the tribulation in which I'm walking.

Maybe you've been there, too. Or perhaps you are there. You feel like you're hopping (or hobbling) from one crisis to the next…

I'm learning firsthand that it's almost impossible to "count things joy" when you're in the middle of the ditch. Yet, later, we can often look back with the perspective of the Kingdom and see, sense, and feel the amazing work that's transformed us into more of who we're destined to be, that image in the mirror.

Though it certainly doesn't look like it in the moment, **something powerful is being produced in you, some sort of diamond of the soul that can only be found in the deepest coal mines of life.**

Think back to Peter's story, the one we referenced in chapter 3. Sinking in the water, denying Jesus, and the other mistakes he made all happened in the context of tough situations. Yet, many of those moments actually refined him so that he was able to walk through the later situations that have come to define him.

You can never reduce a person simply to a label of what they did, any more than you can reduce a book to a simple stack of 26 letters placed in in random order. Nothing makes sense apart from the entire story being threaded together.

We're far more complicated than the raw material and seemingly random episodes of our lives. No one's story should ever be judged by one page, by one chapter, or even by entire sections of their Book of Life.

As my friend David Robinson says, "Do not judge my story by the chapter you walked in on."

Indeed.

Besides, your story is still be written, right?

Your story doesn't excuse you, but it does explain you. And some of the greatest explanations about you to you comes when you embrace the tough stuff and walk through it.

That said, here's an easy way to test your emotional wholeness. Here's the goal, anyway...

EASY AS 1-2-3

There are three items on our Emotional Wholeness Checklist:

- Recognize

- Realize

- Respond

Let's walk through them...

First, *recognize* the emotions you experience.

Remember, there aren't good emotions or bad emotions- just emotions. The more of them we can recognize, the better we can read the temperature around us.

One day during a counseling session I was provided a similar picture to the one below. It lists dozens of feelings. You might find it helpful to read through the list, so that you have an awareness of what some of the feelings are. That might help you tangibly recognize them when you sense them.

HOW MANY FEELINGS CAN YOU RECOGNIZE?

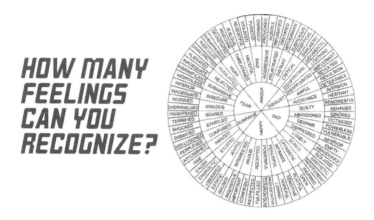

The book *Emotional Intelligence 2.0* reminds us, "Emotions always serve a purpose."[20]

Recognizing them is vital to understanding their purpose. And recognizing requires that we spend some time learning what some of those emotions actually are, so that we can read them properly when we encounter them.

Second, *realize* what your emotions are telling you- *without reacting to them*.

Remember some of the analogies we've made in this book:

---

[20] *Emotional Intelligence 2.0*, Travis Bradberry & Jean Graves, Kindle Version, location 400.

- **Emotions are to the soul what physical pain is to the body**. In the same way physical sensations of pain and pleasure alert us to what's happening in our body, emotional joy and pain- and everything else- tell us the climate of our soul.

- **Emotions are like thermometers.** They don't control us; they simply provide us with valuable information (thermostats set the temperature; thermometers simply read the temperature).

If you can learn to recognize the emotion and then read what it's saying *without* first reacting, you'll find you're light years ahead of 99% of the people in the world around you.

Third, finally, *respond* in a healthy way. After taking in what you sense, and after getting clarity on how you should respond (with intentionality, whatever that response happens to be), then move forward with clarity and humility.

Emotional Wholeness involves recognizing your emotions, reading what they say before you react, and then responding to the world around you in a healthy + intentional way.

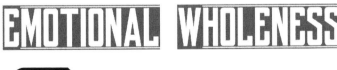

1. RECOGNIZE YOUR EMOTIONS
2. REALIZE WHAT THEY SAY
3. RESPOND IN A HEALTHY WAY

I know. It's way easier said than done. Especially, because... well... our emotions are involved, right?

EMOTIONS IN REAL LIFE

Here's what our "checklist" looks like in the real world:

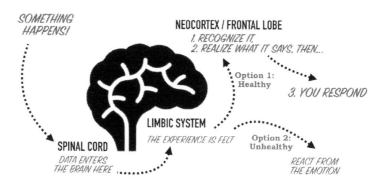

ARE YOU IN CONTROL OF THE EMOTIONS OR ARE THEY IN CONTROL OF YOU?

Let's discuss this graphic briefly, as it will help you in real life situations.

First, something happens (far left of picture). It might be new information that we gather, a phone call or text that is received, or something someone else does.

Second, experience is *felt*. The data then enters our brain (via the spinal cord) and the experience is first *felt* (via the limbic system).

Then, after we *feel* the experience (yes, this happens before we logically think about how to respond!), we have two choices…

- **Option 1: Healthy** = we can work through the Emotional Wholeness Checklist (recognize what you're feeling, realize what it's communicating, then respond in a health way).

- **Option 2: Unhealthy** = react immediately from raw emotion.

Remember, as we discussed in chapter 2, our emotions are one of the "parts" of our whole being. And, like that chain, we'll only be as strong as our weakest link. A more emotionally whole you is a far healthier you- in every area.

5. THE CHECKLIST

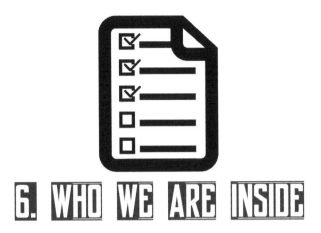

6. WHO WE ARE INSIDE

MAIN IDEA= THE EMOTIONAL WHOLENESS CHECKLIST EMPOWERS YOU TO DEAL WITH NEW SITUATIONS & THE CORRESPONDING FEELINGS IN THE MOMENT. BUT, SOMETIMES YOU NEED TO GO BACK IN ORDER TO MOVE AHEAD.

I'll be honest. I almost deleted this chapter from the book. The goal of this series is to create short books that you can actually read in one sitting, and this bit promised to add about ten more pages. Nonetheless, it's here. I opted to leave it because the info in it is super-super-important and it relates to one of the most valuable yet often-overlooked oils in Young Living's Feelings Kit.

Now, I'm not one for digging up every bit of dirt from the past, finding a demon under every rock, or unearthing every possible traumatic event that may have ever occurred. But I'm not in favor of blasting forward without acknowledging that we're a product of our past, either. **Sometimes- not all the time- it's helpful**

to look back in order to live forward. Especially if our past continues dominating our present.

Let me explain…

One of our adopted sons participated in intensive therapy for almost four years. He was just five when the sessions began.

For the majority of that long season we were involved in meetings with his therapist, Cindi. We joined her for an hour every other Friday morning, followed by an hour with him and her together.

Within the first few months she told us, "There's a little boy and a big boy. The little one is deep inside, hidden. He's the one that is scared and afraid, yet is capable of receiving love. That's the boy he *really* is."

LITTLE ME & BIG ME

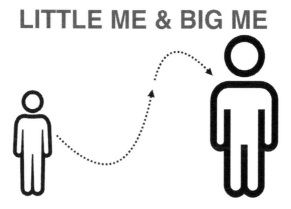

She continued, "But you also have the big boy. That's the fella you're bumping into most of the time. That's the one you're having behavioral issues with. He's been created- *as a projection-* in order to make sure the little boy remains protected, that the little boy gets his needs met."[21]

"Does he have some sort of multiple personality disorder or schizophrenia?" I asked.

"That's a good question," Cindi replied. "No. He doesn't. **On some level we all do this. We have the person we really, truly are that's deep inside of us. Then we have the person we present to the world.** For some people that true self is buried deep. A second self, a false self, has been created as a means of self-protection, generally as a result of trauma."

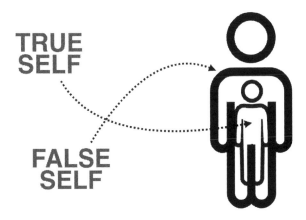

TRUE SELF

FALSE SELF

Cindi explained that when young kids face trauma they often bury the emotionally vulnerable side of themselves deep inside. Adults can do it, too, particularly when

---

21 See Donald Miller's book *Scary Close*, p201. He uses the same analogy that Cindi, our therapist used. Donald makes several other correlations. He says the "big" version seeks applause, while the "little" self seeks intimacy. And the "big" version wants to interact with the many (read: anonymous crowds like you see from the stage or meet via social media), whereas the "little" version craves sharing life with the few.

faced with a traumatic, life-changing event which causes them to feel like the world is no longer a safe place to expose themselves. Even then the roots usually go pretty far back.

Some of this is healthy. God gave us the ability to guard our hearts- not so we would hide them forever, but so that we could deal with pain and protect ourselves from harm in healthy ways (see Proverbs 4:23). Of course, we're not supposed to protect ourselves from *everything*; we're supposed to protect ourselves from *the wrong things* while revealing ourselves to the right things.

The problem is that it's easy to get confused as to what's safe and what's not. When the "safe" things (like family, friends, church) suddenly become unsafe, we tend to self protect from *everything*.

Enter the tough exterior, a massive full-body mask we wear.

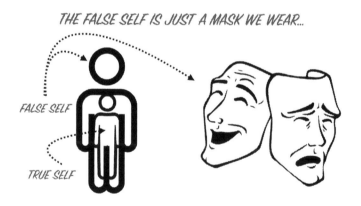

THE FALSE SELF IS JUST A MASK WE WEAR...

FALSE SELF

TRUE SELF

"War heroes play the tough guy, even though they may be dealing with PTSD," Cindi told me. "Rape victims may shift into hyper-activism. Victims of divorce or abandonment may grow an emotionally cold heart- even as they regurgitate the latest things they've read in a book about emotional healing and present themselves as emotionally whole. A lot of the terms people toss out… words like *boundaries*, *gas-lighting*, and other hot-words… people have *no idea* what they really mean. It's all self-protection, something projected in order to hide the hurt and defend themselves. Strangers and acquaintances *think* they look healthy on the outside, but true friends- *if they have any*- know that they're not."[22]

Cindi described how our son spent his first years in Africa. We knew his story well. Since he was so young when the trauma occurred, he had little recollection of many of the events which marked him. We told her most of his story based on the fragments we pieced together. He experienced things like-

- **Rejection & abandonment.** His mom died when he was 18 months old. He lived with his grandparents, who left him and his then 4-year old brother to fend for themselves during the day.

- **Lack.** They never had enough to eat; he constantly felt hungry.

- **Used**. He was sexually abused before his fifth birthday…

He experienced trauma upon trauma. It's no wonder we experienced behavioral issues with him. What person would those life events alone- *at any age*- not scar?

THE LITTLE ME = THE TRUE SELF

His inner child, the small boy inside, was wounded. He projected a larger-than-life external shell- a person that performed well, people-pleased, and presented

---

22 Remember what we discussed in chapter 3- about the two things that help you transform into healthy. The second… was healthy relationships, one in which people have the right to tell you what you need to hear, not just what you want to hear. Without this kind of voice in your life, you'll never grow into the best version of you. We desperately it!

perfectly to the world around him. Well, he presented himself perfectly for a while. Then, in time, those emotional defects became obvious.

Problem was… well… *there was still a little boy living inside.*

"The little boy inside is the true self," Cindi reminded us. "And that little boy is the path to healing. He's got to learn to turn off the outer persona…"

As Cindi taught me about my son during those parenting sessions, it dawned on me that I had an inner self, too- an inner child. Because of things I faced in the past (though nothing like my boy faced) I also created an outer shell.

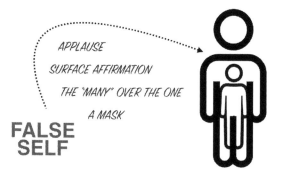

In fact, this is something most of us do.In his memoir about his own inner healing journey, *Scary Close,* Donald Miller talks about his outer self. This outer shell, he writes, is "all theater."[23] That is, it's just a show. It's a show that seeks applause and affirmation and the praise of the "many" instead of intimacy with just a few… all in the name of getting our needs met, of filling some emotional void we haven't learned to deal with.

---

23 See page 21 of his book.

That false self is incapable of giving or receiving love, as it's just a mirage. Like a shadow, it's just an image thrown from a real person onto the world around them:

- Shadows can't connect.

- Shadows can't love.

- Shadows can't heal.

Often, the outer self develops an "Ace" card, something we can lean into that makes us lovable. It might be the way we dress, the hobbies we espouse, or the affinity groups with whom we identify.

Again, **the false self can't receive love, nor can it give it. It can't walk in life and wholeness because, well, it's fake.** And that means it can't carry the weight of your calling, because shadows can't carry *anything*.

For years, I've propped on my shadow to do my bidding for me...

- Much of my teaching... just the persona.

- A lot of what I've written... again, the shadow.

- Some of my social media posts... yeah, just the image... a way to get a "like" and feel instantly validated.

The path forward, for me, isn't to lean into the persona. Or to heal the persona. **You can't heal an image or shadow, you can only heal the true self**. And that comes when the true self finds its complete identity deep inside, as the person we were created to be- from beholding that image we talked about in chapter 3, as well as from walking with wise people who continue calling forth that greatness out of us.

As a kid, my outer self became a fake Christian, someone with a Puritanical moral compass (you'll see the irony of this after you read more of my story), who used good manners and personal charm to present themselves favorably to the world.[24] I kept myself reasonably well-groomed (except for the long season during which I desperately sought significance through work-achievement and allowed my physical self to go, ballooning to over 50 pounds heavier than I am now). I used my above-average athletic skill and my higher-than-normal IQ to fuel the engine of the madness.

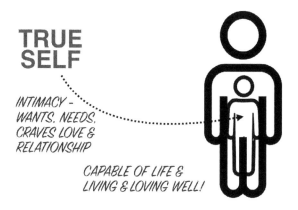

TRUE SELF

*INTIMACY -
WANTS, NEEDS,
CRAVES LOVE &
RELATIONSHIP*

*CAPABLE OF LIFE &
LIVING & LOVING WELL!*

I looked great on the outside. Inside, I struggled.

Over the past few years, the disconnect between the inner child ("Little Andy") and outer self ("Big Andrew") became more obvious. My wife and close friends reminded me that I was adored by my Heavenly Father- that I didn't have to present a false front. I was accepted, just as I am.

---

24 By the way, this shift *can* happen in adulthood. Often, though, the seeds are planted- many times through seemingly insignificant situations- when we are young. Dark stories like mine most often begin as the normal stuff of life happens. We're each the products of living with imperfect people interacting in an imperfect world. Our parents, friends, teachers, ministers, and community leaders all interact with us out of their hurts and wounds, too.

Cristy reminded me that the way in which I view my boys is the way in which Father God sees me. Specifically, she looked at our five-year old.

"Salter is your Little Andy," she told me. "You would do anything in the world for him. And he just wants to be with you. The way you beam when you see him… and the way he rushes to simply sit with you, climb on you, or hang from your arms… that's what your Heavenly Father wants. That's how He sees you."

The goal isn't to "not grow up," nor do we need to crucify our outer self. Rather, **the goal is for the two- the inner and the outer- to become the same, that is, for us to live on the outside the same as we are on the inside.**

FULLY INTEGRATED = HEALTHY, WHOLE

Remember, when we're unhealthy, the outer self is simply smoke and mirrors. Pageantry. A shadow.

On the other hand, when we live in a healthy place, the inner "child" and the outer "man" closely resemble each other.

I know. It's easier said than done. Especially because we live in a world where shadows and images are cast all around us. And especially because we're actually created to enjoy many of the things with which I've struggled…

- We're created for connection.

- We're created- by God- to walk in abundance instead of lack.

- We're created to share our gifts and abilities with others.

The problem, then, isn't that we have these desires. The problem comes when we offer them from the false self rather than offering them from an internal self that's been made whole.

The good news is that we can change. Or, more accurately, the Spirit can do the work of transformation in us.

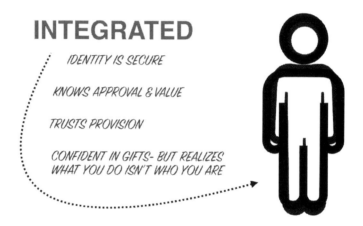

INTEGRATED

IDENTITY IS SECURE

KNOWS APPROVAL & VALUE

TRUSTS PROVISION

CONFIDENT IN GIFTS- BUT REALIZES WHAT YOU DO ISN'T WHO YOU ARE

One way to do this is to go back and work through the Emotional Wholeness Checklist for any past traumatic events you have. This, then, empowers you to recognize where you've reacted with a false outer self instead of responded from the inner self.

When that happens, the "true you" and the "persona" that we've shared with the world become one. We become fully integrated and more totally alive.

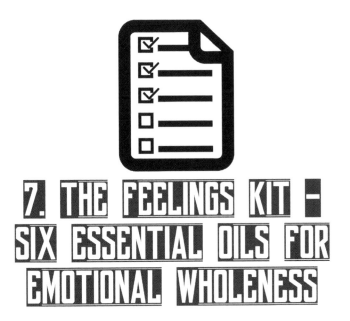

7. THE FEELINGS KIT – SIX ESSENTIAL OILS FOR EMOTIONAL WHOLENESS

MAIN IDEA= USE THE YOUNG LIVING FEELINGS KIT 2X A DAY FOR 30 DAYS (MORNING AND NIGHT), VALIDATING YOUR EMOTIONS AS YOU DO. WITHIN 30 DAYS YOU'LL SEE + SENSE THE WORLD DIFFERENTLY.

Psychologists estimate that 90%+ of our decisions are made from our feelings instead of our thoughts. It's easy to confuse the two.

Since you've looked at the Emotional Wholeness Checklist, you know how to respond in a healthy way that involves your thoughts instead of simply reacting from your feelings- thereby **allowing your feelings to serve you rather than being tossed by them.**

Remember, feelings aren't bad. They're gifts. They've been given to us by the Creator to help us understand what's happening around us and what's happening to us. In the same way which physical sensations can communicate joy, pain, tiredness, soreness, energy and dozens of other things to us, so also can our feelings.

The problem is… well, if we don't know *how* to recognize them… then we might make decisions from them without being aware.

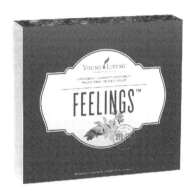

Enter the Feelings Kit from YL (item #312508), a boxed set of six essential oils- each chosen because of its ability to enhance your overall emotional well-being.

We'll work through the Emotional Wholeness Checklist for each. Remember the steps-

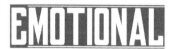 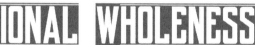

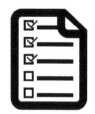

1. RECOGNIZE YOUR EMOTIONS
2. REALIZE WHAT THEY SAY
3. RESPOND IN A HEALTHY WAY

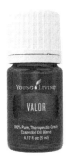

Valor = courage to face whatever + however. Was inspired by a blend Roman soldiers used before going into combat.

Apply to the soles of your feet.

- **Recognize**- the difficulty of the situation you are facing.

- **Realize**- acknowledge your fear, apprehension, uncertainty (or any other emotion you are feeling about that situation). Courage (read: Valor) isn't the absence of tribulation; it's a feeling of bravery that honestly assesses the situation and chooses to walk through it with a humble confidence.

- **Respond**- with courage. Courage (read: Valor) isn't the absence of tribulation; it's a feeling of bravery that honestly assesses the situation and chooses to walk through it with a humble confidence.

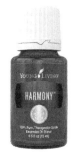

Harmony = to bring things back in balance. To give you confidence + creativity.

Apply to your heart.

- **Recognize**- the trials and tribulations you are facing, admitting that some things aren't as they're designed to be or how you hoped they would be. This might be a relational issue, a struggle at work, or even something in your physical body.

- **Realize**- the disconnect between what's happening and what you hoped would happen.

- **Respond**- and acknowledge that where you are in life never determines "who you are." Your identity and your value as a person are secure, regardless of any circumstance you face.

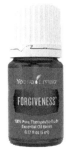

Forgiveness = the key to unlocking freedom.

Apply to your stomach, your gut (which is your "second brain") as you forgive and let go of things you need to leave behind.

- **Recognize**- where and why you may feel hurt because of something someone has said or done, no matter how large or how small it may be.

- **Realize**- that unforgiveness "holds us hostage" to them and what they've done, and that forgiving them doesn't equate with saying that what they've done is right or OK... rather, forgiveness acknowledges that whatever happened was 1) wrong, yet 2) we're releasing the burden of punishing them, resolving their behavior, or creating an outcome that we can control. We entrust it to God.

- **Respond**- by reminding yourself, when feelings about the situation surface, that you were hurt by their actions, but that you've forgiven them and entrusted the results to the Lord. You may need to consistently remind yourself that you've set it in the Lord's hands and off-loaded that burden.

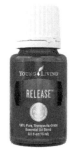

Release = b/c negative energy actually goes into your blood and streams through your body, feeding your cells.

Apply to your wrists, at the pulse points and visualize yourself letting go of negative thoughts.

- **Recognize**- that life is tough, that you may be carrying burdens because of various situations in which you've found yourself. These could be situations you created, or they could be the result of just being in the "wrong place at the wrong time." Further, the situation could be something "bad" or it could be just the normal course of life. Often, noise and chatter and long to-do lists can burden us.

- **Realize**- that you need to let those things go, whatever they are. As you apply the oil to your wrists, visualize yourself letting go of the weight.

   (Whereas forgiveness deals with a relational issue between people, release most often refers to situations.)

- **Respond**- as you move forward, reminding yourself that you have let that burden go. Sure, you may encounter the same situation again… but, remind yourself that this one has been released…

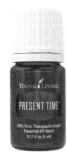

Present Time = b/c we want to live in the moment. Not in the past. Not in the future. Here.

Apply a few drops to your chest and neck as you "face forward" in your day.

- **Recognize**- that something may be pulling you to a different time and place. It could be feelings of worry about the past or anxiety about the future (or even something else).

- **Realize**- that the only place in which you can live is right here, right now. There is nothing you can do about past happenings, and the future things you are worried about aren't here yet. You will deal with them when they are "present."

  (It may prove helpful to release some of those things.)

- **Respond**- by centering yourself here and now. Commit to the next best step, whether it be going to the office, spending time with your kids, reading a book… whatever it is, commit to being fully present in that moment, regardless of how late or small it seems to be.

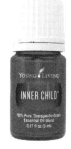

Inner Child = b/c living your best life is a matter of awakening to who you truly are, the greatness you were created with in the beginning!

Apply to the back of your waist, near your spine + the back of your neck.

- **Recognize**- that there may be a "false self" which you're projecting to the world around you (review chapter 6). Discern why you are doing that- whether you're seeking approval from others, whether you're feeling lonely and disconnected, whether you have the need to be noticed… or even something else.

- **Realize**- that you are more than enough. You've been "wonderfully made" (Psalm 139:14), with an incredible destiny that was scripted for you before time began (Ephesians 2:8-10).

- **Respond**- with a sense of gratitude that you need only be the person you are designed to be, that you are enough.

USING THE FEELINGS KIT

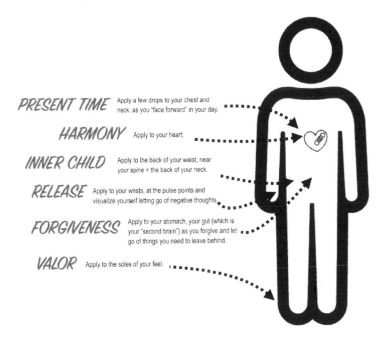

PRESENT TIME — Apply a few drops to your chest and neck. as you "face forward" in your day.

HARMONY — Apply to your heart.

INNER CHILD — Apply to the back of your waist, near your spine + the back of your neck.

RELEASE — Apply to your wrists, at the pulse points and visualize yourself letting go of negative thoughts.

FORGIVENESS — Apply to your stomach, your gut (which is your "second brain") as you forgive and let go of things you need to leave behind.

VALOR — Apply to the soles of your feet.

****

Tip = For best results, use the oils twice a day (at morning + night). Do so for 30 days. Applying them will take you less than 5 minutes to do and you'll reap powerful results!

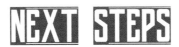

NEXT STEPS

Now, you need to acquire the tools to get started. We suggest you order Young Living's Premium Starter Kit (it's an amazing value- it comes with 12 essential oils, a diffuser, and several other items!). You will eventually want the *Feelings Kit*, too.

If you're able to acquire these at the same time, do so! If not, order the Premium Starter Kit right away- and set an Essential Rewards order for the *Feelings Kit* to come to you next month. (Essential Rewards is a non-obligation, non-contract program that gives you discounted shipping and points back which you can use for free products. We don't buy anything unless we do it on this program- we love free stuff!).

If you're waiting to get the *Feelings Kit* (you'll want to order the other kit *first*, so that you receive the 24% discount on the *Feelings Kit*!), place it on Essential Rewards now and it will ship in approximately 30 days, giving you time to learn the first set of oils. (By placing the order on Essential Rewards, you earn points towards future *free* products!)

To place your order, consult with the person who gave you this material if they are a business-building distributor with Young Living Essential Oils. You will need their coupon code to receive the wholesale discount!

If they are not a distributor OR if you found this info on your own, *please go to* facebook.com/OilyApp *and send a PM, or connect through Instagram @OilyApp.*

ABOUT OILYAPP PLUS

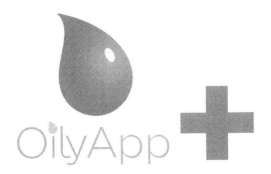

Want to watch the videos of this script? And other videos?

Oily App plus was created for you!

OilyApp+ is a web-based monthly membership / subscription service which provides you with each of the following:

- A monthly class- including a downloadable script AND the videos for the material in this book

- Graphics to match the class!

- 60 second videos to review each of the products mentioned in the class

- Access to Diamond+ leaders and biz-building tips

CLASSES
= Monthly video + script for you to watch and use on your own!

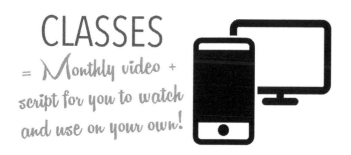

Here's a deeper dive on each of these features!

Monthly Feature #1 = An online class you can use to encourage, equip, and empower your team!

Every month- generally, the second week of the month- we go live and teach a class. Here's where it gets good… OilyApp+ subscribers receive forever access to the recording of that class, AS WELL AS the downloadable PDF or script we use.

GRAPHICS
= Our best graphics and copy sent straight to Plus! members

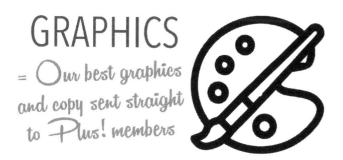

Join the class simply to learn, or take advantage of the info by passing it on to others!

Monthly Feature #2 = Our best graphics available for you to download + share!

We've pulled the best graphics and multi-pic posts from our Instagram feed and placed them where you can download them, then re-use them to share with prospects and grow your business. And, we've included our swipe copy in the files. Use it, edit it, whatever- it's there for you.

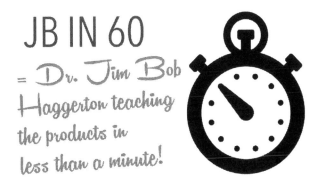

JB IN 60
= Dr. Jim Bob Haggerton teaching the products in less than a minute!

Monthly Feature #3 = How'd you like Dr. Jim Bob Haggerton to teach you about the products?! Done!

Specifically, he'll do it in 60 seconds or less. Whatever products we review in our class- be it the Oils of the Bible, the PSK, the core supplements... he'll give you the 60 second overview of each!

BIZ TIPS
= Videos + more to encourage, equip, and empower you to grow

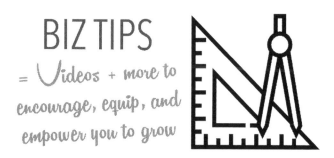

In the online portal, you can login and watch + re-watch as many times as you'd like!

Monthly feature #4 = A recorded video call with one of the top leaders in Young Living! How would you like to hear how one Royal Crown Diamond hit the top rank without ever hosting a class- just by working through social media? Or, how would you like to learn how another did it WITHOUT social media?

LEADERS
= Exclusive access to top leaders teaching from their wheelhouse!

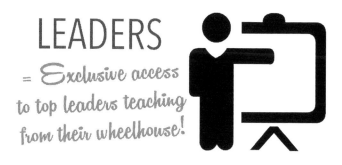

What about learning leadership, work-family balance, gaining momentum, or finding your passion form others?

Each month we feature a recorded convo from one of the top leaders teaching from their unique wheelhouse.

Monthly Feature #5 = Bonus videos and other tools we've created to make the biz super-simple and pleasantly practical!

You wouldn't dream of going to work somewhere without understanding how you get paid, and what you can do to make the most of your time. Somehow, we stumble into network marketing and forget to step back and ask those same questions, though.

Each month, we'll drop a resource about the comp plan, about teaching the business, or some other aspect that encourages, equips, and empowers YOU to reach your potential!

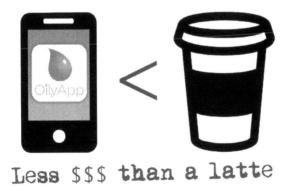

Less $$$ than a latte

You can find all of this our on website- www.OilyApp.com!

And, it's affordable. In fact, it all costs you less than a latte!

The Feelings Kit from Young Living is something I use just about every single day. Sometimes I use it twice- in the morning AND at night, after the morning shower AND before I go to bed...

In fact, I've got a routine I use with it. After discussing the "what" and "why" of emotions I walk you through it.

In this book, too, I outline 3 simple steps (yes, they're EASIER said than done, for sure) that will empower you to allow your emotions to serve you RATHER THAN you being held hostage by them, yanked around by them...

Our emotions are gifts, things God gave us in order to help us understand what's happening around us and in us. In the same way that physical sensations such as pleasure and pain help us encounter the world, so also do emotional sensations (such as fear and joy).

And, no, Fear isn't a liar. It can serve you. And serve you well. As can all of your emotions. The "good" ones, the "bad" ones, and everything in between.

In fact, your total health will never rise above the level of your emotional wholeness. So, flip the page. Let's get this one right and allow our emotions to empower us rather than enslave us!

Made in the USA
Columbia, SC
13 January 2020